Simply Keto Diet

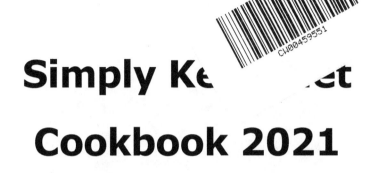

Cookbook 2021

Best Cookbook With Practical

Ketogenic Recipes for Heal Body

and Lose Weight Fast

Tanya Scofield

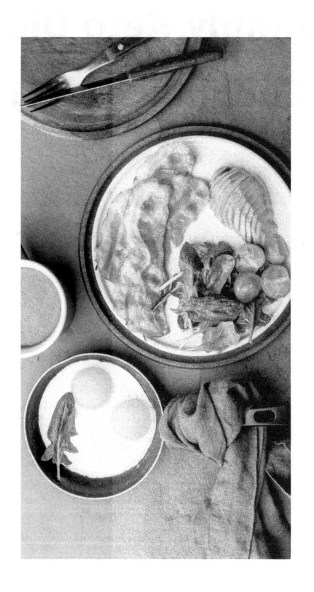

Table of Contents

INTRODUCTION 8

BREAKFAST 13

CHICKEN CORDON BLEU WITH CAULIFLOWER 13
SESAME-CRUSTED TUNA WITH GREEN BEANS 15
ROSEMARY ROASTED PORK WITH CAULIFLOWER 17
GRILLED SALMON AND ZUCCHINI WITH MANGO SAUCE 19
BEEF AND BROCCOLI STIR-FRY 22
PARMESAN-CRUSTED HALIBUT WITH ASPARAGUS 24
HEARTY BEEF AND BACON CASSEROLE 26
SESAME WINGS WITH CAULIFLOWER 28
FRIED COCONUT SHRIMP WITH ASPARAGUS 30
CREAMY QUESO DIP 32
COCONUT CHICKEN CURRY WITH CAULIFLOWER RICE 34
PUMPKIN SPICED ALMONDS 36
TZATZIKI DIP WITH CAULIFLOWER 38
CLASSIC GUACAMOLE DIP 40
EASY SKILLET PANCAKES 42
KETO EVERYTHING BAGELS 44
TURMERIC CHICKEN AND KALE SALAD WITH FOOD, LEMON AND
HONEY 47
OVERNIGHT "NOATS" 50
QUICK KETO BLENDER MUFFINS 52
BACON APPETIZERS 54
BUCKWHEAT SPAGHETTI WITH CHICKEN CABBAGE AND SAVORY
FOOD RECIPES IN MASS SAUCE 55
FROZEN KETO COFFEE 58
ASIAN KING JUMPED JAMP 60
BUCKWHEAT PASTA SALAD 62
GREEK SALAD SKEWERS 64
ANTIPASTI SKEWERS 67
KALE, EDAMAME AND TOFU CURRY 69
CHOCOLATE CUPCAKES WITH MATCHA ICING 71
SESAME CHICKEN SALAD 73
JALAPENO POPPERS 75
BLT PARTY BITES 77
STRAWBERRIES AND CREAM SMOOTHIE 79
CAULI FLITTERS 81

Bacon Wrapped Chicken Breast 83
No-Bake Keto Power Bars 85
Avocado Toast 88
Almond Flour Pancakes 90
Chicken Avocado Egg Bacon Salad 92
Keto Flu Combat Smoothie 94
Bacon Hash 96
Egg Salad 98
Bagels with Cheese 100
Capicola Egg Cups 101
Scrambled Eggs 102
Frittata with Spinach 104
Cheese Omelet 105

LUNCH **106**

Buttered Cod 106
Salmon with Red Curry Sauce 108
Salmon Teriyaki 110
Pesto Shrimp with Zucchini Noodles 112

CONCLUSION **115**

The information in the following pages is broadly considered a truthful and accurate account of facts and as such, any inattention, use, or misuse of the information in question by the reader will render any resulting actions solely under their purview. There are no scenarios in which the publisher or the original author of this work can be in any fashion deemed liable for any hardship or damages that may befall them after undertaking information described herein.

Additionally, the information in the following pages is intended only for informational purposes and should thus be thought of as universal. As befitting its nature, it is presented without assurance regarding its prolonged validity or interim quality. Trademarks that are mentioned are done without written consent and can in no way be considered an endorsement from the trademark holder.

INTRODUCTION

So the Ketogenic Diet is all about reducing the amount of carbohydrates you eat. Does this mean you won't get the kind of energy you need for the day? Of course not! It only means that now, your body has to find other possible sources of energy. Do you know where they will be getting that energy? Even before we talk about how to do keto – it's important to first consider why this particular diet works. What actually happens to your body to make you lose weight? As you probably know, the body uses food as an energy source. Everything you eat is turned into energy, so that you can get up and do whatever you need to accomplish for the day. The main energy source is sugar so what happens is that you eat something, the body breaks it down into sugar, and the sugar is processed into energy. Typically, the "sugar" is taken directly from the food you eat so if you eat just the right amount of food, then your body is fueled for the whole day. If you eat too much, then the sugar is stored in your body – hence the accumulation of fat.

But what happens if you eat less food? This is where the Ketogenic Diet comes in. You see, the process of creating sugar from food is usually faster if the food happens to be rich in carbohydrates. Bread, rice, grain, pasta – all of these are carbohydrates and they're the easiest food types to turn into energy.

So here's the situation – you are eating less carbohydrates every day. To keep you energetic, the body breaks down the stored fat and turns them into molecules called ketone bodies. The process of turning the fat into ketone bodies is called "Ketosis" and obviously – this is where the name of the Ketogenic Diet comes from. The ketone bodies take the place of glucose in keeping you energetic. As long as you keep your carbohydrates reduced, the body will keep getting its energy from your body fat.

The Ketogenic Diet is often praised for its simplicity and when you look at it properly, the process is really straightforward. The Science behind the effectivity of the diet is also well-documented, and has been proven multiple times by different medical fields. For example, an article on Diet Review by Harvard provided a lengthy discussion on how the Ketogenic Diet works and why it is so effective for those who choose to use this diet.

But Fat Is the Enemy...Or Is It?

No – fat is NOT the enemy. Unfortunately, years of bad science told us that fat is something you have to avoid – but it's actually a very helpful thing for weight loss! Even before we move forward with this book, we'll have to discuss exactly what "healthy fats" are, and why they're actually the good guys. To do this, we need to make a distinction between the different kinds of fat. You've probably heard of them before and it is a little bit confusing at first. We'll try to go through them as simply as possible:

Saturated fat. This is the kind you want to avoid. They're also called "solid fat" because each molecule is packed with hydrogen atoms. Simply put, it's the kind of fat that can easily cause a blockage in your body. It can raise cholesterol levels and lead to heart problems or a stroke. Saturated fat is something you can find in meat, dairy products, and other processed food items. Now, you're probably wondering: isn't the Ketogenic Diet packed with saturated fat? The answer is: not necessarily. You'll find later in the recipes given that the Ketogenic Diet promotes primarily unsaturated fat or healthy fat. While there are definitely many meat recipes in the list, most of these recipes contain healthy fat sources.

Unsaturated Fat. These are the ones dubbed as healthy fat. They're the kind of fat you find in avocado, nuts, and other ingredients you usually find in Keto-friendly recipes. They're known to lower blood cholesterol and actually come in two types: polyunsaturated and monounsaturated. Both are good for your body but the benefits slightly vary, depending on what you're consuming.

BREAKFAST

Chicken Cordon Bleu with Cauliflower

Preparation Time: 10 minutes

Cooking Time: 45 minutes

Servings: 4

Ingredients:

- 4 boneless chicken breast halves (about 12 ounces)
- 4 slices deli ham
- 4 slices Swiss cheese
- 1 large egg, whisked well
- 2 ounces pork rinds
- ¼ cup almond flour
- ¼ cup grated parmesan cheese
- ½ teaspoon garlic powder
- Salt and pepper
- 2 cups cauliflower florets

Directions:

1. Preheat the oven to 350 ° F and add a foil on a baking sheet.

2. Sandwich the breast half of the chicken between parchment parts and pound flat.
3. Spread the bits out and cover with ham and cheese sliced over.
4. Roll the chicken over the fillings and then dip into the beaten egg.
5. In a food processor, mix the pork rinds, almond flour, parmesan, garlic powder, salt and pepper,
6. And pulse into fine crumbs.
7. Roll the rolls of chicken in the mixture of pork rind then put them on the baking sheet.
8. Throw the cauliflower into the baking sheet with the melted butter and fold.
9. Bake for 45 minutes until the chicken is fully cooked.

Nutrition: Calories: 420 Fats: 23 Protein: 7 Carbohydrates: 0

Sesame-Crusted Tuna with Green Beans

Preparation Time: 15 minutes
Cooking Time: 5 minutes
Servings: 4
Ingredients:

- ¼ cup white sesame seeds
- ¼ cup black sesame seeds
- 4 (6-ounce) ahi tuna steaks
- Salt and pepper
- 1 tablespoon olive oil
- 1 tablespoon coconut oil
- 2 cups green beans

Directions:

1. In a shallow dish, mix the two kinds of sesame seeds.
2. Season the tuna with pepper and salt.
3. Dredge the tuna in a mixture of sesame seeds.
4. Heat up to high heat the olive oil in a skillet, then add the tuna.
5. Cook for 1 to 2 minutes until it turns seared, then sear on the other side.
6. Remove the tuna from the skillet, and let the tuna rest while using the coconut oil to heat the skillet.

---

7. Fry the green beans in the oil for 5 minutes then use sliced tuna to eat.

Nutrition: Calories: 420 Fats: 23 Protein: 7 Carbohydrates: 0

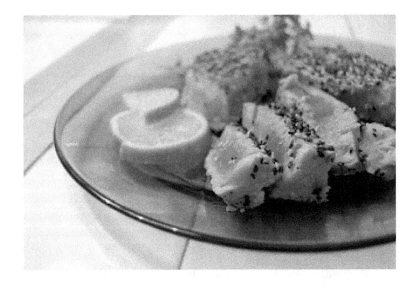

Rosemary Roasted Pork with Cauliflower

Preparation Time: 10 minutes

Cooking Time: 20 minutes

Servings: 4

Ingredients:

- 1 ½ pounds boneless pork tenderloin
- 1 tablespoon coconut oil
- 1 tablespoon fresh chopped rosemary
- Salt and pepper
- 1 tablespoon olive oil
- 2 cups cauliflower florets

Directions:

1. Rub the coconut oil into the pork, then season with the rosemary, salt, and pepper.
2. Heat up the olive oil over medium to high heat in a large skillet.
3. Add the pork on each side and cook until browned for 2 to 3 minutes.
4. Sprinkle the cauliflower over the pork in the skillet.
5. Reduce heat to low, then cover the skillet and cook until the pork is cooked through for 8 to 10 minutes.

6. Slice the pork with cauliflower and eat.

Nutrition: Calories: 320 Fats: 37 Protein: 3
Carbohydrates: 1

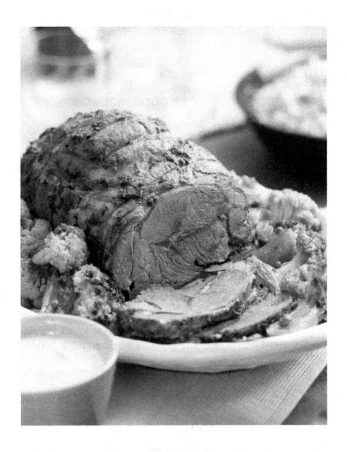

Grilled Salmon and Zucchini with Mango Sauce

Preparation Time: 5 minutes
Cooking Time: 10 minutes
Servings: 4
Ingredients:

- 4 (6-ounce) boneless salmon fillets
- 1 tablespoon olive oil
- Salt and pepper
- 1 large zucchini, sliced in coins
- 2 tablespoons fresh lemon juice
- ½ cup chopped mango
- ¼ cup fresh chopped cilantro
- 1 teaspoon lemon zest
- ½ cup canned coconut milk

Directions:

1. Preheat a grill pan to heat, and sprinkle with cooking spray liberally.
2. Brush with olive oil to the salmon and season with salt and pepper.
3. Apply lemon juice to the zucchini, and season with salt and pepper.
4. Put the zucchini and salmon fillets on the grill pan.

5. Cook for 5 minutes then turn all over and cook for another 5 minutes.
6. Combine the remaining ingredients in a blender and combine to create a sauce.
7. Serve the side-drizzled salmon filets with mango sauce and zucchini.

Nutrition: Calories: 350 Fats: 23 Protein: 7 Carbohydrates: 6

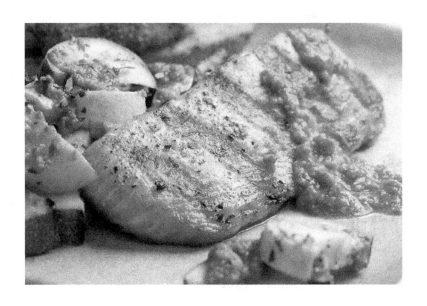

Beef and Broccoli Stir-Fry

Preparation Time: 20 minutes

Cooking Time: 15 minutes

Servings: 4

Ingredients:

- ¼ cup soy sauce
- 1 tablespoon sesame oil
- 1 teaspoon garlic chili paste
- 1-pound beef sirloin
- 2 tablespoons almond flour
- 2 tablespoons coconut oil
- 2 cups chopped broccoli florets
- 1 tablespoon grated ginger
- 3 cloves garlic, minced

Directions:

1. In a small bowl, whisk the soy sauce, sesame oil, and chili paste together.
2. In a plastic freezer bag, slice the beef and mix with the almond flour.
3. Pour in the sauce and toss to coat for 20 minutes, then let rest.
4. Heat up the oil over medium to high heat in a large skillet.

5. In the pan, add the beef and sauce and cook until the beef is browned.
6. Move the beef to the skillet sides, then add the broccoli, ginger, and garlic.
7. Sauté until tender-crisp broccoli, then throw it all together and serve hot.

Nutrition: Calories: 350 Fats: 19 Protein: 37 Carbohydrates: 6

Parmesan-Crusted Halibut with Asparagus

Preparation Time: 10 minutes

Cooking Time: 15 minutes

Servings: 4

Ingredients:

- 2 tablespoons olive oil
- ¼ cup butter, softened
- Salt and pepper
- ¼ cup grated Parmesan
- 1-pound asparagus, trimmed
- 2 tablespoons almond flour
- 4 (6-ounce) boneless halibut fillets
- 1 teaspoon garlic powder

Directions:

1. Preheat the oven to 400 F and line a foil-based baking sheet.
2. Throw the asparagus in olive oil and scatter over the baking sheet.
3. In a blender, add the butter, Parmesan cheese, almond flour, garlic powder, salt and pepper, and mix until smooth.
4. Place the fillets with the asparagus on the baking sheet, and spoon the Parmesan over the eggs.

5. Bake for 10 to 12 minutes, then broil until browned for 2 to 3 minutes.

Nutrition: Calories: 415 Fats: 26 Protein: 42 Carbohydrates: 3

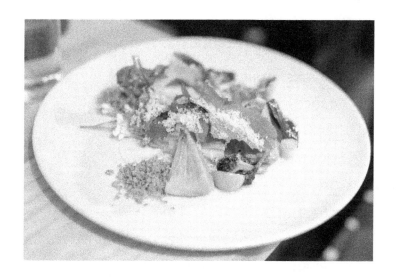

Hearty Beef and Bacon Casserole

Preparation Time: 25 minutes

Cooking Time: 30 minutes

Servings: 8

Ingredients:

- 8 slices uncooked bacon
- 1 medium head cauliflower, chopped
- ¼ cup canned coconut milk
- Salt and pepper
- 2 pounds ground beef (80% lean)
- 8 ounces mushrooms, sliced
- 1 large yellow onion, chopped
- 2 cloves garlic, minced

Direction:

1. Preheat to 375 F on the oven.
2. Cook the bacon in a skillet until it crispness, then drain and chop on paper towels.
3. Bring to boil a pot of salted water, then add the cauliflower.
4. Boil until tender for 6 to 8 minutes then drain and add the coconut milk to a food processor.
5. Mix until smooth, then sprinkle with salt and pepper.

6. Cook the beef until browned in a pan, then wash the fat away.
7. Remove the mushrooms, onion, and garlic, then move to a baking platter.
8. Place on top of the cauliflower mixture and bake for 30 minutes.
9. Broil for 5 minutes on high heat, then sprinkle with bacon to serve.

Nutrition: Calories: 410 Fats: 25 Protein: 37 Carbohydrates: 6

Sesame Wings with Cauliflower

Preparation Time: 5 minutes

Cooking Time: 30 minutes

Servings: 4

Ingredients:

- 2 ½ tablespoons soy sauce
- 2 tablespoons sesame oil
- 1 ½ teaspoons balsamic vinegar
- 1 teaspoon minced garlic
- 1 teaspoon grated ginger
- Salt
- 1-pound chicken wing, the wings itself
- 2 cups cauliflower florets

Directions:

1. In a freezer bag, mix the soy sauce, sesame oil, balsamic vinegar, garlic, ginger, and salt, then add the chicken wings.
2. Coat flip, then chill for 2 to 3 hours.
3. Preheat the oven to 400 F and line a foil-based baking sheet.
4. Spread the wings along with the cauliflower onto the baking sheet.
5. Bake for 35 minutes, then sprinkle on to serve with sesame seeds.

Nutrition: Calories: 400 Fats: 15 Protein: 5 Carbohydrates: 3

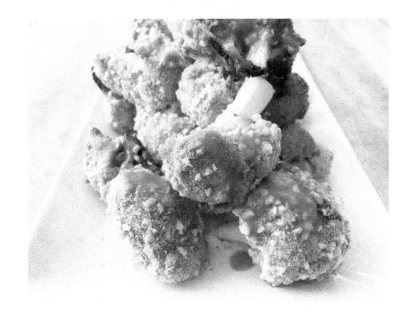

Fried Coconut Shrimp with Asparagus

Preparation Time: 15 minutes

Cooking Time: 10 minutes

Servings: 6

Ingredients:

- 1 ½ cups shredded unsweetened coconut
- 2 large eggs
- Salt and pepper
- 1 ½ pounds large shrimp, peeled and deveined
- ½ cup canned coconut milk
- 1-pound asparagus, cut into 2-inch pieces

Directions:

1. Pour the coconut onto a shallow platter.
2. Beat the eggs in a bowl with a little salt and pepper.
3. Dip the shrimp into the egg first, then dredge with coconut.
4. Heat up coconut oil over medium-high heat in a large skillet.
5. Add the shrimp and fry over each side for 1 to 2 minutes until browned.
6. Remove the paper towels from the shrimp and heat the skillet again.

7. Remove the asparagus and sauté to tender-crisp with salt and pepper, then serve with the shrimp.

Nutrition: Calories: 535 Fats: 38 Protein: 16 Carbohydrates: 3

Creamy Queso Dip

Preparation Time: 15 minutes

Cooking Time: 5 minutes

Servings: 8

Ingredients:

- 4 ounces chorizo, crumbled
- 1 clove garlic, minced
- ¼ cup heavy cream
- 6 ounces shredded white cheddar cheese
- 2 ounces shredded pepper jack cheese
- ¼ teaspoon xanthan gum
- Pinch salt
- 1 jalapeno, seeded and minced
- 1 small tomato, diced

Directions:

1. Cook the chorizo in a skillet until browned evenly, then scatter in a dish.
2. At medium-low heat, pressure the skillet and add the garlic–cook for 30 seconds.
3. Stir in the heavy cream, then add the cheese a little at a time, stirring frequently until it melts.
4. Sprinkle with salt and xanthan gum, then mix well, and cook until thickened.

5. Add the tomato and jalapeno, then serve, dipping with vegetables.

Nutrition: Calories: 195 Fats: 16 Protein: 12

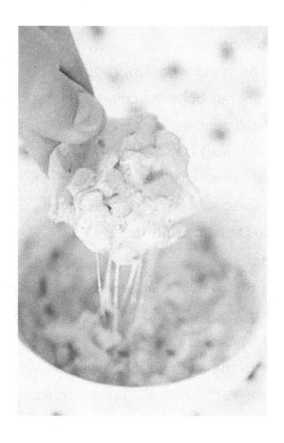

Coconut Chicken Curry with Cauliflower Rice

Preparation Time: 15 minutes

Cooking Time: 30 minutes

Servings: 6

Ingredients:

- 1 tablespoon olive oil
- 1 medium yellow onion, chopped
- 1 ½ pounds boneless chicken thighs, chopped
- Salt and pepper
- 1 (14-ounce) can coconut milk
- 1 tablespoon curry powder
- 1 ¼ teaspoon ground turmeric
- 3 cups riced cauliflower

Directions:

1. Heat the oil over medium heat, in a large skillet.
2. Add the onions, and cook for about 5 minutes, until translucent.
3. Stir in the chicken and season with salt and pepper-cook for 6 to 8 minutes, stirring frequently until all sides are browned.
4. Pour the coconut milk into the pan, then whisk in the curry and turmeric powder.

5. Simmer until hot and bubbling, for 15 to 20 minutes.
6. Meanwhile, steam the cauliflower rice until tender with a few tablespoons of water.
7. Serve the cauliflower rice over the curry.

Nutrition: Calories: 430 Fats: 29 Protein: 9 Carbohydrates: 3

Pumpkin Spiced Almonds

Preparation Time: 5 minutes

Cooking Time: 25 minutes

Servings: 4

Ingredients:

- 1 tablespoon olive oil
- 1 ¼ teaspoon pumpkin pie spice
- Pinch salt
- 1 cup whole almonds, raw

Direction:

1. Preheat the oven to 300 ° F, and line a parchment baking sheet.
2. In a mixing bowl, whisk together the olive oil, pumpkin pie spice, and salt.
3. Toss in the almonds until coated evenly, then scatter onto the baking sheet.
4. Bake and place in an airtight container for 25 minutes then cool down completely.

Nutrition: Calories: 170 Fats: 15 Protein: 5 Carbohydrates: 3

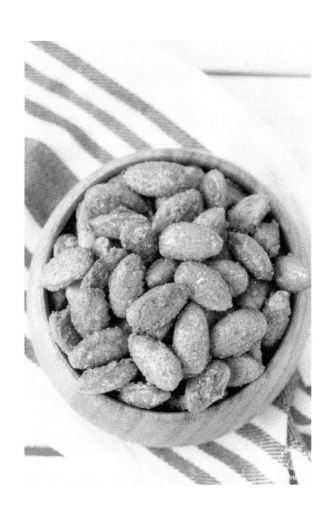

Tzatziki Dip with Cauliflower

Preparation Time: 10 minutes

Cooking Time: 0 minutes

Servings: 6

Ingredients:

- ½ (8-ounce) package cream cheese, softened
- 1 cup sour cream
- 1 tablespoon ranch seasoning
- 1 English cucumber, diced
- 2 tablespoons chopped chives
- 2 cups cauliflower florets

Directions:

1. Use an electric mixer to pound the cream cheese until smooth.
2. Stir in the sour cream and ranch seasoning, beat until smooth.
3. Fold in the cucumbers and chives, then chill with cauliflower florets for dipping before serving.

Nutrition: Calories: 125 Fats: 10 Protein: 5 Carbohydrates: 3

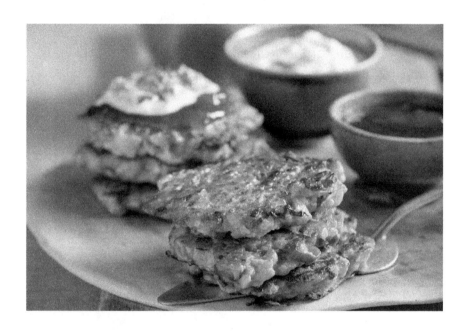

Classic Guacamole Dip

Preparation Time: 15 minutes

Cooking Time: 0 minutes

Servings: 4

Ingredients:

- 2 mediums avocado, pitted
- 1 small yellow onion, diced
- 1 small tomato, diced
- ¼ cup fresh chopped cilantro
- 1 tablespoon fresh lime juice
- 1 jalapeno, seeded and minced
- 1 clove garlic, minced
- Salt
- Sliced veggies to serve

Directions:

1. Mash avocado flesh into a bowl.
2. Stir the onion, tomato, cilantro, lime juice, garlic, and jalapeno in a bowl
3. Season lightly with salt and spoon into a bowl – serve with sliced veggies.

Nutrition: Calories: 225 Fats: 20 Protein: 12 Carbohydrates: 3

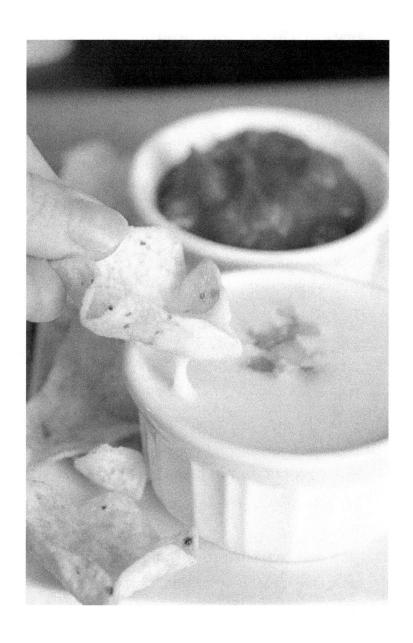

Easy Skillet Pancakes

Preparation Time: 5 minutes

Cooking Time: 5 minutes

Servings: 8

Ingredients:

- 8 ounces cream cheese
- 8 eggs
- 2 tablespoons coconut flour
- 2 teaspoons baking powder
- 1 teaspoon ground cinnamon
- ½ teaspoon vanilla extract
- 1 teaspoon liquid stevia or sweetener of choice (optional)
- 2 tablespoons butter

Directions

1. In a blender, combine the cream cheese, eggs, coconut flour, baking powder, cinnamon, vanilla, and stevia (if using). Blend until smooth.

2. In a large skillet over medium heat, melt the butter.

3. Use half the mixture to pour four evenly sized pancakes and cook for about a minute, until you see bubbles on top. Flip the pancakes and cook for another minute. Remove from the pan and

add more butter or oil to the skillet if needed. Repeat with the remaining batter.

4. Top with butter and eat right away, or freeze the pancakes in a freezer-safe resealable bag with sheets of parchment in between, for up to 1 month.

Nutrition: Calories: 179 Total Fat: 15g Protein: 8g Total Carbs: 3g Fiber: 1g Net Carbs: 2g

Keto Everything Bagels

Preparation Time: 10 minutes

Cooking Time: 15 minutes

Servings: 8

Ingredients:

- 2 cups shredded mozzarella cheese
- 2 tablespoons labneh cheese (or cream cheese)
- 1½ cups almond flour
- 1 egg
- 2 teaspoons baking powder
- ¼ teaspoon sea salt
- 1 tablespoon

Directions

1. Preheat the oven to 400ºF.
2. In a microwave-safe bowl, combine the mozzarella and labneh cheeses. Microwave for 30 seconds, stir, then microwave for another 30 seconds. Stir well. If not melted completely, microwave for another 10 to 20 seconds.
3. Add the almond flour, egg, baking powder, and salt to the bowl and mix well. Form into a dough using a spatula or your hands.
4. Cut the dough into 8 roughly equal pieces and form into balls.

5. Roll each dough ball into a cylinder, then pinch the ends together to seal.

6. Place the dough rings in a nonstick donut pan or arrange them on a parchment paper–lined baking sheet.

7. Sprinkle with the seasoning and bake for 12 to 15 minutes or until golden brown.

8. Store in plastic bags in the freezer and defrost overnight in the refrigerator. Reheat in the oven or toaster for a quick grab-and-go breakfast.

Nutrition: Calories: 241 Total Fat: 19g Protein: 12g Total Carbs: 5.5g Fiber: 2.5g Net Carbs: 3g

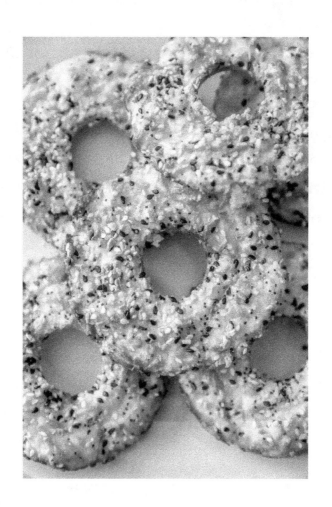

Turmeric Chicken and Kale Salad with Food, Lemon and Honey

Preparation Time: 20 minutes

Cooking Time: 15 minutes

Servings: 4

Ingredients:

- For the chicken:
- 1 teaspoon of clarified butter or 1 tablespoon of coconut oil
- ½ medium brown onion, diced
- 250-300 g / 9 ounces minced chicken meat or diced chicken legs
- 1 large garlic clove, diced
- 1 teaspoon of turmeric powder
- 1 teaspoon of lime zest
- ½ lime juice
- ½ teaspoon of salt + pepper
- For the salad:
- 6 stalks of broccoli or 2 cups of broccoli flowers
- 2 tablespoons of pumpkin seeds (seeds)
- 3 large cabbage leaves, stems removed and chopped
- ½ sliced avocado
- Handful of fresh coriander leaves, chopped

- Handful of fresh parsley leaves, chopped
- For the dressing:
- 3 tablespoons of lime juice
- 1 small garlic clove, diced or grated
- 3 tablespoons of virgin olive oil (I used 1 tablespoon of avocado oil and 2 tablespoons of EVO)
- 1 teaspoon of raw honey
- ½ teaspoon whole or Dijon mustard
- ½ teaspoon of sea salt with pepper

Directions:

1. Heat the coconut oil in a pan. Add the onion and sauté over medium heat for 4-5 minutes, until golden brown. Add the minced chicken and garlic and stir 2-3 minutes over medium-high heat, separating.

2. Add your turmeric, lime zest, lime juice, salt and pepper, and cook, stirring consistently, for another 3-4 minutes. Set the ground beef aside.

3. While your chicken is cooking, put a small saucepan of water to the boil. Add your broccoli and cook for 2 minutes. Rinse with cold water and cut into 3-4 pieces each.

4. Add the pumpkin seeds to the chicken pan and toast over medium heat for 2 minutes, frequently stirring to avoid burning. Season with a little salt.

Set aside. Raw pumpkin seeds are also good to use.

5. Put the chopped cabbage in a salad bowl and pour it over the dressing. Using your hands, mix, and massage the cabbage with the dressing. This will soften the cabbage, a bit like citrus juice with fish or beef Carpaccio: it "cooks" it a little.

6. Finally, mix the cooked chicken, broccoli, fresh herbs, pumpkin seeds, and avocado slices.

Nutrition: 232 calories Fat 11 Fiber 9 Carbs 8 Protein 14

Overnight "noats"

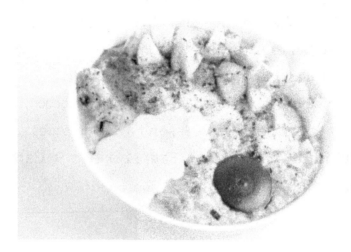

Preparation Time: 5 minutes plus overnight to chill

Cooking Time: 10 minutes

Servings: 1

Ingredients:

- 2 tablespoons hulled hemp seeds
- 1 tablespoon chia seeds
- ½ scoop (about 8 grams) collagen powder
- ½ cup unsweetened nut or seed milk (hemp, almond, coconut, and cashew)

Direction:

1. In a small mason jar or glass container, combine the hemp seeds, chia seeds, collagen, and milk.
2. Secure tightly with a lid, shake well, and refrigerate overnight.

Nutrition: Calories: 263 Total Fat: 19g Protein: 16g Total Carbs: 7g Fiber: 5g Net Carbs: 2g

Quick Keto Blender Muffins

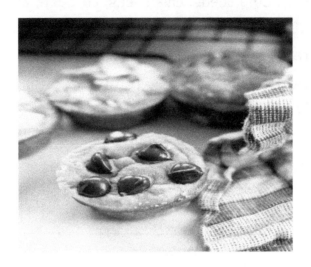

Preparation Time: 5 minutes

Cooking Time: 25 minutes

Servings: 12

Ingredients

- Butter, ghee, or coconut oil for greasing the pan
- 6 eggs
- 8 ounces cream cheese, at room temperature
- 2 scoops flavored collagen powder
- 1 teaspoon ground cinnamon
- 1 teaspoon baking powder
- Few drops or dash sweetener (optional)

Directions:

1. Preheat the oven to 350ºF. Grease a 12-cup muffin pan very well with butter, ghee, or coconut oil. Alternatively, you can use silicone cups or paper muffin liners.

2. In a blender, combine the eggs, cream cheese, collagen powder, cinnamon, baking powder, and sweetener (if using). Blend until well combined and pour the mixture into the muffin cups, dividing equally.

3. Bake for 22 to 25 minutes until the muffins are golden brown on top and firm.

4. Let cool then store in a glass container or plastic bag in the refrigerator for up to 2 weeks or in the freezer for up to 3 months.

5. To Servings refrigerated muffins, heat in the microwave for 30 seconds. To Servings from frozen, thaw in the refrigerator overnight and then microwave for 30 seconds, or microwave straight from the freezer for 45 to 60 seconds or until heated through.

Nutrition: Calories: 120 Total Fat: 10g Protein: 6g Total Carbs: 1.5g Fiber: 0g Net Carbs: 1.5g

Bacon Appetizers

Preparation Time: 15 minutes

Cooking Time: 2 hours

Servings: 6

Ingredients:

- 1 pack Keto crackers
- ¾ cup Parmesan cheese, grated
- 1 lb. bacon, sliced thinly

Directions:

1. Preheat your oven to 250 degrees F.
2. Arrange the crackers on a baking sheet.
3. Sprinkle cheese on top of each cracker.
4. Wrap each cracker with the bacon.
5. Bake in the oven for 2 hours.

Nutrition: Calories 440 Total Fat 33.4g Saturated Fat 11g Cholesterol 86mg Sodium 1813mg Total Carbohydrate 3.7g Dietary Fiber 0.1g Total Sugars 0.1g Protein 29.4g Potassium 432mg

Buckwheat Spaghetti with Chicken Cabbage and Savory Food Recipes in Mass Sauce

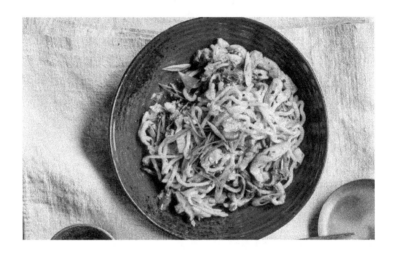

Preparation Time: 15 minutes
Cooking Time: 15 minutes'
Servings: 2
Ingredients:

- For the noodles:
- 2-3 handfuls of cabbage leaves (removed from the stem and cut)
- Buckwheat noodles 150g / 5oz (100% buckwheat, without wheat)

- 3-4 shiitake mushrooms, sliced
- 1 teaspoon of coconut oil or butter
- 1 brown onion, finely chopped
- 1 medium chicken breast, sliced or diced
- 1 long red pepper, thinly sliced (seeds in or out depending on how hot you like it)
- 2 large garlic cloves, diced
- 2-3 tablespoons of Tamari sauce (gluten-free soy sauce)
- For the miso dressing:
- 1 tablespoon and a half of fresh organic miso
- 1 tablespoon of Tamari sauce
- 1 tablespoon of extra virgin olive oil
- 1 tablespoon of lemon or lime juice
- 1 teaspoon of sesame oil (optional)

Directions:

1. Boil a medium saucepan of water. Add the black cabbage and cook 1 minute, until it is wilted. Remove and reserve, but reserve the water and return to boiling. Add your soba noodles and cook according to the directions on the package (usually about 5 minutes). Rinse with cold water and reserve.

2. In the meantime, fry the shiitake mushrooms in a little butter or coconut oil (about a teaspoon) for

2-3 minutes, until its color is lightly browned on each side. Sprinkle with sea salt and reserve.

3. In that same pan, heat more coconut oil or lard over medium-high heat. Fry the onion and chili for 2-3 minutes, and then add the chicken pieces. Cook 5 minutes on medium heat, stirring a few times, then add the garlic, tamari sauce, and a little water. Cook for another 2-3 minutes, stirring continuously until your chicken is cooked.

4. Finally, add the cabbage and soba noodles and stir the chicken to warm it.

5. Stir the miso sauce and sprinkle the noodles at the end of the cooking, in this way you will keep alive all the beneficial probiotics in the miso.

Nutrition: 305 calories Fat 11 Fiber 7 Carbs 9 Protein 12

Frozen keto coffee

Preparation Time: 5 minutes

Cooking Time: 20 minutes

Servings: 1

Ingredients:

- 12 ounces coffee, chilled
- 1 scoop MCT powder (or 1 tablespoon MCT oil)
- 1 tablespoon heavy (whipping) cream
- Pinch ground cinnamon
- Dash sweetener (optional)
- ½ cup ice

Directions:

1. In a blender, combine the coffee, MCT powder, cream, cinnamon, sweetener (if using), and ice. Blend until smooth.

Nutrition: Calories: 127; Total Fat: 13g; Protein: 1g; Total Carbs: 1.5g; Fiber: 1g; Net Carbs: 0.5g

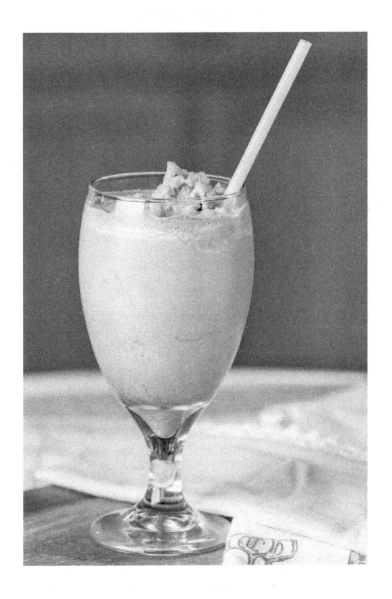

Asian King Jumped Jamp

Preparation Time: 15 minutes

Cooking Time: 10 minutes

Servings: 4

Ingredients:

- 150 g / 5 oz. of raw shelled prawns, not chopped
- Two teaspoons of tamari (you can use soy sauce if you don't avoid gluten)
- Two teaspoons of extra virgin olive oil
- 75 g / 2.6 oz. soba (buckwheat pasta)
- 1 garlic clove, finely chopped
- 1 bird's eye chili, finely chopped
- 1 teaspoon finely chopped fresh ginger.
- 20 g / 0.7 oz. of sliced red onions
- 40 g / 1.4 oz. of celery, cut and sliced
- 75 g / 2.6 oz. of chopped green beans
- 50 g / 1.7 oz. of chopped cabbage
- 100 ml / ½ cup of chicken broth
- 5 g celery or celery leaves

Directions:

1. Heat a pan over high heat, and then cook the prawns in 1 teaspoon of tamari and 1 teaspoon of oil for 2-3 minutes. Transfer the prawns to a

plate. Clean the pan with kitchen paper as it will be reused.

2. Cook your noodles in boiling water for 5-8 minutes or as indicated on the package. Drain and set aside.

3. Meanwhile, fry the garlic, chili and ginger, red onion, celery, beans, and cabbage in the remaining oil over medium-high heat for 2-3 minutes. Add your broth and allow it to boil, and then simmer for a minute or two, until the vegetables are cooked but crunchy.

4. Add shrimp, noodles and celery/celery leaves to the pan, bring to a boil again, then remove from the heat and serve.

Nutrition: Calories 223 Protein 34 Fat 2 Carbs 6

Buckwheat Pasta Salad

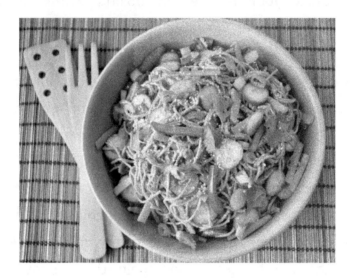

Preparation Time: 10 minutes

Cooking Time: 30 minutes

Servings: 4

Ingredients:

- 50 g / 1.7 oz. buckwheat pasta
- Large handful of rockets
- A small handful of basil leaves
- Eight cherry tomatoes halved
- 1/2 avocado, diced
- Ten olives
- 1 tablespoon. extra olive virgin oil

- 20 g / 0.70 oz. pine nuts

Directions:

1. Combine all the ingredients except your pine nuts. Arrange your combination on a plate, and then scatter the pine nuts over the top.

Nutrition: 125 calories Fat 6 Fiber 5 Carbs 10 Protein 11

Greek Salad Skewers

Preparation Time: 35 minutes

Cooking Time: 0 minutes

Servings: 2

Ingredients:

- Two wooden skewers, soaked in water for 30 minutes before use
- Eight large black olives
- Eight cherry tomatoes
- 1 yellow pepper, cut into eight squares.
- ½ red onions, you can cut in half and separated into eight pieces
- 100 g / 3.5 oz. (about 10cm) cucumber, cut into four slices and halved
- 100 g / 3.5 oz. feta, cut into eight cubes
- For the dressing:
- 1 tablespoon. extra olive virgin oil
- Juice of ½ lemons
- 1 teaspoon. of your balsamic vinegar
- ½ clove garlic, ensure it peeled and crushed
- Basil leaves chopped (or ½ teaspoon. dried mixed herbs to replace basil and oregano)
- Oregano leaves,
- Salt and grounded black pepper

Directions:

1. Blend each skewer with the salad ingredients in the order
2. Put all your dressing ingredients into a bowl and mix thoroughly. Pour over the skewers.

Nutrition: Calories 99 Protein 34 Fat 4 Carbs 5

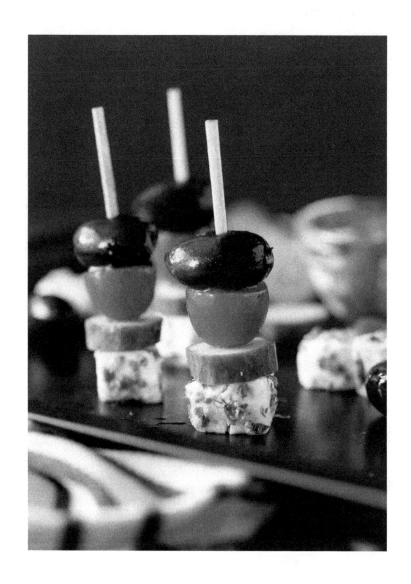

Antipasti Skewers

Preparation Time: 10 minutes

Cooking Time: 0 minute

Servings: 6

Ingredients:

- 6 small mozzarella balls
- 1 tablespoon olive oil
- Salt to taste
- 1/8 teaspoon dried oregano
- 2 roasted yellow peppers, sliced into strips and rolled
- 6 cherry tomatoes
- 6 green olives, pitted
- 6 Kalamata olives, pitted
- 2 artichoke hearts, sliced into wedges
- 6 slices salami, rolled
- 6 leaves fresh basil

Directions:

1. Toss the mozzarella balls in olive oil.
2. Season with salt and oregano.
3. Thread the mozzarella balls and the rest of the ingredients into skewers.
4. Serve in a platter.

Nutrition: Calories 180 Total Fat 11.8g Saturated Fat 4.5g Cholesterol 26mg Sodium 482mg Total Carbohydrate 11.7g Dietary Fiber 4.8g Total Sugars 4.1g Protein 9.2g Potassium 538mg

Kale, Edamame and Tofu Curry

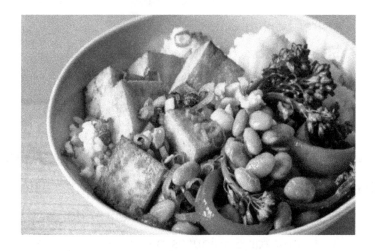

Preparation Time: 20 minutes

Cooking Time: 40 minutes

Servings: 3

Ingredients:

- 1 tablespoon rapeseed oil
- 1 large onion, chopped
- Four cloves garlic, peeled and grated
- 1 large thumb (7cm) fresh ginger, peeled and grated
- 1 red chili, deseeded and thinly sliced
- 1/2 teaspoon ground turmeric
- 1/4 teaspoon cayenne pepper
- 1 teaspoon paprika
- 1/2 teaspoon ground cumin

- 1 teaspoon salt
- 250 g / 9 oz. dried red lentils
- 1-liter boiling water
- 50 g / 1.7 oz. frozen soya beans
- 200 g / 7 oz. firm tofu, chopped into cubes
- Two tomatoes, roughly chopped
- Juice of 1 lime
- 200 g / 7 oz. kale leaves stalk removed and torn

Directions:

1. Put the oil in a pan over low heat. Add your onion and cook for 5 minutes before adding the garlic, ginger, and chili and cooking for a further 2 minutes. Add your turmeric, cayenne, paprika, cumin, and salt and Stir through before adding the red lentils and stirring again.

2. Pour in the boiling water and allow it to simmer for 10 minutes, reduce the heat and cook for about 20-30 minutes until the curry has a thick '•porridge' consistency.

3. Add your tomatoes, tofu and soya beans and cook for a further 5 minutes. Add your kale leaves and lime juice and cook until the kale is just tender.

Nutrition: Calories 133 Carbohydrate 54 Protein 43

Chocolate Cupcakes with Matcha Icing

Preparation Time: 35 minutes

Cooking Time: 0 minutes

Servings: 4

Ingredients:

- 150g / 5 oz. self-rising flour
- 200 g / 7 oz. caster sugar
- 60 g / 2.1 oz. cocoa
- ½ teaspoon. salt
- ½ teaspoon. fine espresso coffee, decaf if preferred
- 120 ml / ½ cup milk
- ½ teaspoon. vanilla extract
- 50 ml / ¼ cup vegetable oil
- 1 egg
- 120 ml / ½ cup of water
- For the icing:
- 50 g / 1.7 oz. butter,
- 50 g / 1.7 oz. icing sugar
- 1 tablespoon matcha green tea powder
- ½ teaspoon vanilla bean paste
- 50 g / 1.7 oz. soft cream cheese

Directions:

1. Heat the oven and Line a cupcake tin with paper

2. Put the flour, sugar, cocoa, salt, and coffee powder in a large bowl and mix well.

3. Add milk, vanilla extract, vegetable oil, and egg to dry ingredients and use an electric mixer to beat until well combined. Gently pour the boiling water slowly and beat on low speed until completely combined. Use the high speed to beat for another minute to add air to the dough. The dough is much more liquid than a normal cake mix. Have faith; It will taste fantastic!

4. Arrange the dough evenly between the cake boxes. Each cake box must not be more than ¾ full. Bake for 15-18 minutes, until the dough resumes when hit. Remove from oven and allow cooling completely before icing.

5. To make the icing, beat your butter and icing sugar until they turn pale and smooth. Add the matcha powder and vanilla and mix again. Add the cream cheese and beat until it is smooth. Pipe or spread on the cakes.

Nutrition: calories435 Fat 5 Fiber 3 Carbs 7 Protein 9

Sesame Chicken Salad

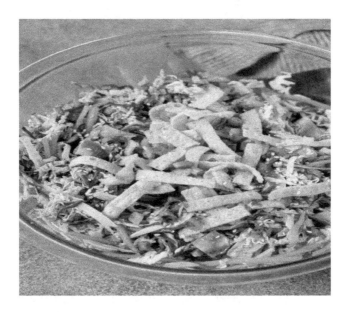

Preparation Time: 20 minutes

Cooking Time: 0 minutes

Servings: 4

Ingredients:

- 1 tablespoon of sesame seeds
- 1 cucumber, peeled, halved lengthwise, without a teaspoon, and sliced.
- 100 g / 3.5 oz. cabbage, chopped
- 60 g pak choi, finely chopped
- ½ red onion, thinly sliced

- Large parsley (20 g / 0.7 oz.), chopped.
- 150 g / 5 oz. cooked chicken, minced
- For the dressing:
- 1 tablespoon of extra virgin olive oil
- 1 teaspoon of sesame oil
- 1 lime juice
- 1 teaspoon of light honey
- 2 teaspoons soy sauce

Directions:

1. Roast your sesame seeds in a dry pan for 2 minutes until they become slightly golden and fragrant.
2. Transfer to a plate to cool.
3. In a small bowl, mix olive oil, sesame oil, lime juice, honey, and soy sauce to prepare the dressing.
4. Place the cucumber, black cabbage, pak choi, red onion, and parsley in a large bowl and mix gently.
5. Pour over the dressing and mix again.
6. Distribute the salad between two dishes and complete with the shredded chicken. Sprinkle with sesame seeds just before serving.

Nutrition: Calories 345 Fat 5 Fiber 2 Carbs 10 Protein 4

Jalapeno Poppers

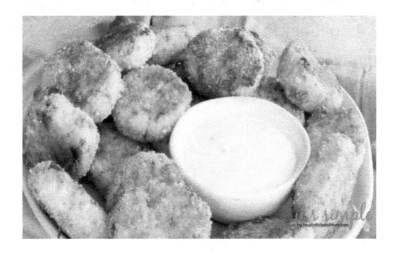

Preparation Time: 30 minutes

Cooking Time: 60 minutes

Servings: 10

Ingredients:

- 5 fresh jalapenos, sliced and seeded
- 4 oz. package cream cheese
- ¼ lb. bacon, sliced in half

Directions:

1. Preheat your oven to 275 degrees F.
2. Place a wire rack over your baking sheet.
3. Stuff each jalapeno with cream cheese and wrap in bacon.
4. Secure with a toothpick.
5. Place on the baking sheet.

6. Bake for 1 hour and 15 minutes.

Nutrition: Calories 103 Total Fat 8.7g Saturated Fat 4.1g Cholesterol 25mg Sodium 296mg Total Carbohydrate 0.9g Dietary Fiber 0.2g Total Sugars 0.3g Protein 5.2g Potassium 93mg

BLT Party Bites

Preparation Time: 35 minutes

Cooking Time: 0 minute

Servings: 8

Ingredients:

- 4 oz. bacon, chopped
- 3 tablespoons panko breadcrumbs
- 1 tablespoon Parmesan cheese, grated
- 1 teaspoon mayonnaise
- 1 teaspoon lemon juice
- Salt to taste
- ½ heart Romaine lettuce, shredded
- 6 cocktail tomatoes

Directions:

1. Put the bacon in a pan over medium heat.
2. Fry until crispy.
3. Transfer bacon to a plate lined with paper towel.
4. Add breadcrumbs and cook until crunchy.
5. Transfer breadcrumbs to another plate also lined with paper towel.
6. Sprinkle Parmesan cheese on top of the breadcrumbs.
7. Mix the mayonnaise, salt and lemon juice.
8. Toss the Romaine in the mayo mixture.

9. Slice each tomato on the bottom to create a flat surface so it can stand by itself.

10. Slice the top off as well.

11. Scoop out the insides of the tomatoes.

12. Stuff each tomato with the bacon, Parmesan, breadcrumbs and top with the lettuce.

Nutrition: Calories 107 Total Fat 6.5g Saturated Fat 2.1g Cholesterol 16mg Sodium 360mg Total Carbohydrate 5.4g Dietary Fiber 1.5g Total Sugars 3.3g Protein 6.5g Potassium 372mg

Strawberries and Cream Smoothie

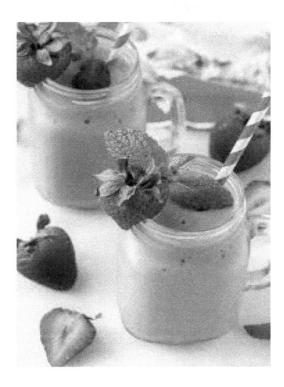

Preparation Time: 5 minutes

Cooking Time: 15 minutes

Servings: 1

Ingredients:

- 5 medium strawberries, hulled
- 3 tablespoons heavy (whipping) cream
- 3 ice cubes
- Your favorite vanilla-flavored sweetener

Directions:

1. In a blender, combine all the ingredients and blend until smooth. Enjoy right away!

Nutrition: Calories: 176 Total Fat: 16g Protein: 2g Total Carbs: 6g Fiber: 1g Net Carbs: 5g

Cauli Flitters

Preparation Time: 10 minutes

Cooking Time: 15 minutes

Servings: 2

Ingredients:

- 2 eggs
- 1 head of cauliflower
- 1 tbsp. yeast
- sea salt, black pepper
- 1-2 tbsp. ghee
- 1 tbsp. turmeric
- 2/3 cup almond flour

Directions:

1. Place the cauliflower into a large pot and start to boil it for 8 mins. Add the florets into a food processor and pulse them.
2. Add the eggs, almond flour, yeast, turmeric, salt and pepper to a mixing bowl. Stir well. Form into patties.
3. Heat your ghee to medium in a skillet. Form your fritters and cook until golden on each side (3-4 mins).
4. Serve it while hot.

Nutrition: Calories: 238 kcal Fat: 23 g Carbs: 5 g Protein: 6 g

Bacon Wrapped Chicken Breast

Preparation Time: 10 minutes

Cooking Time: 45 minutes

Servings: 4

Ingredients

- 4 boneless, skinless chicken breast
- 8 oz. sharp cheddar cheese
- 8 slices bacon
- 4 oz. sliced jalapeno peppers
- 1 tsp garlic powder
- Salt and pepper to taste

Directions

1. Preheat the oven at around 3500F. Ensure to season both sides of chicken breast well with salt, garlic powder, and pepper. Place the chicken breast on a non-stick baking sheet (foil-covered). Cover the chicken with cheese and add jalapeno slices. Cut the bacon slices in half and then place the four halves over each piece of chicken. Bake for around 30 to 45 minutes at most. If the chicken is set but the bacon still feels undercooked, you may want to put it under the broiler for a few minutes. Once done, serve hot

with a side of low carb garlic parmesan roasted asparagus.

Nutrition: Calories: 640 Fat: 48g Carbohydrates: 6g Fiber: 3g Net carbs: 3g Protein: 47g

No-Bake Keto Power Bars

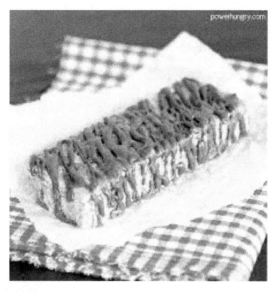

Preparation Time: 10 Minutes plus Overnight to Chill

Cooking Time: 20 minutes

Servings: 12 bars

Ingredients:

- ½ cup pili nuts
- ½ cup whole hazelnuts
- ½ cup walnut halves
- ¼ cup hulled sunflower seeds
- ¼ cup unsweetened coconut flakes or chips
- ¼ cup hulled hemp seeds
- 2 tablespoons unsweetened cacao nibs

- 2 scoops collagen powder (I use 1 scoop Perfect Keto vanilla collagen and 1 scoop Perfect Keto unflavored collagen powder)
- ½ teaspoon ground cinnamon
- ½ teaspoon sea salt
- ¼ cup coconut oil, melted
- 1 teaspoon vanilla extract
- Stevia or monk fruit to sweeten (optional if you are using unflavored collagen powder)

Directions:

1. Line a 9-inch square baking pan with parchment paper.
2. In a food processor or blender, combine the pili nuts, hazelnuts, walnuts, sunflower seeds, coconut, hemp seeds, cacao nibs, collagen powder, cinnamon, and salt and pulse a few times.
3. Add the coconut oil, vanilla extract, and sweetener (if using). Pulse again until the ingredients are combined. Do not over pulse or it will turn to mush. You want the nuts and seeds to still have some texture.
4. Pour the mixture into the prepared pan and press it into an even layer. Cover with another piece of parchment (or fold over extra from the first piece)

and place a heavy pan or dish on top to help press the bars together.

5. Refrigerate overnight and then cut into 12 bars. Store the bars in individual storage bags in the refrigerator for a quick grab-and-go breakfast.

Nutrition: Calories: 242 Total Fat: 22g Protein: 6.5g Total Carbs: 4.5g Fiber: 2.5g Net Carbs: 2g

Avocado Toast

Preparation Time: 20 minutes

Cooking Time: 40 minutes

Servings: 2

Ingredients

- ½ cup grass-fed butter
- 2 tbsp coconut oil
- 7 large eggs
- 1 tsp baking powder
- 2 cups almond flour
- ½ tsp xanthan gum
- ½ tsp kosher salt
- 1 medium avocado

Directions

1. Preheat over at 3500F. Beat eggs for around two minutes with a mixer at high speed. Then, add coconut oil and butter (both melted) to the eggs and continue beating. Ensure that oil and butter are not too warm to cook the eggs. Add remaining bread ingredients and mix well. Now, the batter should become thick. Pour batter in a non-stick loaf pan lined with parchment paper. Let it bake for 45 minutes or until the fork comes clean through the middle.

2. For topping, toast two slices of your keto bread to your liking. Slice the whole avocado thinly, without the skin or pit. Use these to make one long strip of overlapping slices. Roll these into a spiral and that is it! Enjoy your keto bread with avocado topping.

Nutrition: Calories: 350 Fat: 32g Carbohydrates: 7g Fiber: 4g Net carbs: 3g Protein: 10g

Almond Flour Pancakes

Preparation Time: 5 minutes

Cooking Time: 5 minutes

Servings: 4

Ingredients

- ½ cup almond flour
- ½ cup cream cheese
- 4 medium eggs
- ½ tsp cinnamon
- ½ tsp granulated sweetener
- 1 tsp grass-fed butter
- 1 tbsp sugar-free syrup

Directions

1. Add all the ingredients into a blender and let them blend in well. Once done, set the batter aside.

2. On a non-stick pan at medium heat, fry pancakes with melted butter. Once the center starts to bubble, turn over. Once done with the pancake, move on to the rest, using the batter.

3. Finally, serve your pancakes warm, along with some low carb fruit or with an exquisite side of sugar-free syrup to enjoy a healthy and tasty breakfast.

Nutrition: Calories: 234 Fat: 20g Carbohydrates: 4g Fiber: 1.5g Net carbs: 2.5g Protein: 11g

Chicken Avocado Egg Bacon Salad

Preparation Time: 10 minutes

Cooking Time: 10 minutes

Servings: 4

Ingredients

- 12 oz. cooked chicken breast
- 6 slices crumbled bacon
- 3 boiled eggs cut into cubes
- 1 cup cherry tomatoes cut into halves
- 1/2 small sliced red onion
- 1 large avocado(s)
- 1/2 stick finely chopped celery
- Salad Dressing
- 1/2 cup olive oil mayonnaise
- 2 tbsp. sour cream
- 1 tsp Dijon mustard
- 4 tbsp. extra virgin olive oil
- 2 cloves minced garlic
- 2 tsp lemon juice
- 4 cups lettuce
- Salt and pepper to taste

Directions

1. Combine all the ingredients together and mix them well for the salad dressing. Then, combine

chicken, tomatoes, bacon, eggs, red onions, and celery together. Add about ¾ of the salad dressing and mix them well. Add the avocado and toss together gently. Check the taste and, if needed, add the remainder of the salad dressing as well. Finally, add salt and pepper to taste and then serve it over lettuce.

Nutrition: Calories: 387 Fat: 27g Carbohydrates: 2.5g Fiber: 1g Net carbs: 1.5g Protein: 24g

Keto Flu Combat Smoothie

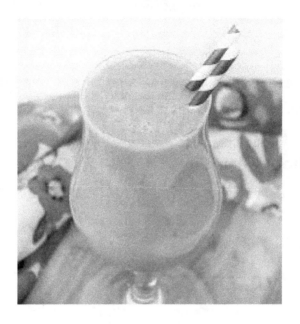

Preparation Time: 5 Minutes

Cooking Time: 15 minutes

Servings: 1

Ingredients:

- ½ cup unsweetened nut or seed milk (hemp, almond, coconut, and cashew)
- 1 cup spinach
- ½ medium avocado (about 75 grams), pitted and peeled
- 1 scoop MCT powder (or 1 tablespoon MCT oil)
- ½ tablespoon unsweetened cacao powder

- ¼ teaspoon of sea salt
- Dash sweetener (optional)
- ½ cup ice

Directions:

1. In a blender, combine the milk, spinach, avocado, MCT powder, cacao powder, salt, sweetener (if using), and ice and blend until smooth.

Nutrition: Calories: 249 Total Fat: 21g Protein: 5g Total Carbs: 10g Fiber: 8g Net Carbs: 2g

Bacon Hash

Preparation Time: 5 minutes

Cooking Time: 10 minutes

Servings: 2

Ingredients:

- Small green pepper (1)
- Jalapenos (2)
- Small onion (1)
- Eggs (4)
- Bacon slices (6)

Directions:

1. Chop the bacon into chunks using a food processor. Set aside for now. Slice the onions and peppers into thin strips. Dice the jalapenos as small as possible.
2. Heat a skillet and fry the veggies. Once browned, combine the fixings and cook until crispy. Place on a serving dish with the eggs.

Nutrition: Carbohydrates: 9 grams Protein: 23 grams Fats: 24 grams Calories: 366

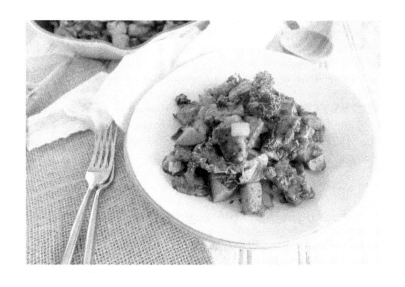

Egg Salad

Preparation Time: 15 minutes

Cooking Time: 10 minutes

Servings: 4

Ingredients

- 6 eggs
- 2 tbsp mayonnaise
- 1 tsp Dijon mustard
- 1 tsp lemon juice
- Salt and pepper to taste

Directions

1. In a medium saucepan, place the solid eggs gently.
2. Add some cold water so that the eggs are covered around an inch. Boil them for around 10 minutes.
3. Once done, remove them from the heat and let them cool. Peel the eggs while running them under cold water. Now add these in a food processor and pulse until they are chopped.
4. Add and stir mayonnaise, lemon juice, mustard, and salt and pepper. Ensure to taste and then adjust as necessary.
5. Finally, serve them with a bit of lettuce leaves and, if needed, bacon for wrapping.

Nutrition: Calories: 222 Fat: 19g Net carbs: 1g
Protein: 13g

Bagels with Cheese

Preparation Time: 10 minutes

Cooking Time: 15 minutes

Servings: 6

Ingredients:

- Mozzarella cheese (2.5 cups)
- Baking powder (1 tsp.)
- Cream cheese (3 oz.)
- Almond flour (1.5 cups)
- Eggs (2)

Directions:

1. Shred the mozzarella and combine with the flour, baking powder, and cream cheese in a mixing container. Pop into the microwave for about one minute. Mix well.

2. Let the mixture cool and add the eggs. Break apart into six sections and shape into round bagels. Note: You can also sprinkle with a seasoning of your choice or pinch of salt if desired.

3. Bake them for approximately 12 to 15 minutes. Serve or cool and store.

Nutrition: Carbohydrates: 8 grams Protein: 19 grams Fats: 31 grams Calories: 374

Capicola Egg Cups

Preparation Time: 5 minutes

Cooking Time: 15 minutes

Servings: 4

Ingredients:

- 8 eggs
- 1 cup cheddar cheese
- 4 oz. capicola or bacon (slices)
- salt, pepper, basil

Directions:

1. Preheat the oven to 400°F. You will need 8 wells of a standard-size muffin pan.
2. Place the slices in the 8 wells, forming a cup shape. Sprinkle into each cup some of the cheese, according to your liking.
3. Crack an egg into each cup, season them with salt and pepper.
4. Bake for 10-15 mins. Serve hot, top it with basil.

Nutrition: Carbs: 1 g Fat: 11 g Protein: 16 g Calories: 171 kcal

Scrambled Eggs

Preparation Time: 2 minutes

Cooking Time: 8 minutes

Servings: 4

Ingredients:

- 4 oz. butter
- 8 eggs
- salt and pepper for taste

Directions:

1. Crack the eggs in a bowl, and whisk them together, while seasoning it.
2. Melt the butter in a skillet over medium heat, but don't turn it into brown.
3. Pour the eggs into the skillet and cook it for 1-2 mins, until they look and feel fluffy and creamy.
4. Tip: If you want to shake things up, you can pair this one up with bacon, salmon, or maybe avocado as well.

Nutrition: Carbs: 1 g Fat: 31 g Protein: 11 g Calories: 327 kcal

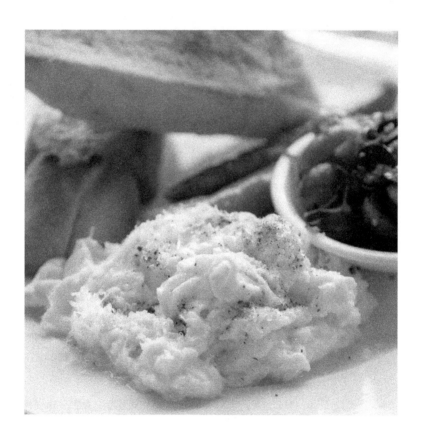

Frittata with Spinach

Preparation Time: 5 minutes

Cooking Time: 30 minutes

Servings: 4

Ingredients:

- 8 eggs
- 8 ozs. fresh spinach
- 5 ozs. diced bacon
- 5 ozs. shredded cheese
- 1 cup heavy whipping cream
- 2 tbsps. butter
- salt and pepper

Directions:

1. Preheat the oven to 350 °F
2. Fry the bacon until crispy, add the spinach and cook until wilted. Set them aside.
3. Whisk the cream and eggs together, and pour it into the baking dish.
4. Add the cheese, spinach, and bacon on the top, and place in the oven. Bake for 25-30 minutes, until golden brown on top.

Nutrition: Carbs: 4 g Fat: 59 g Protein: 27 g Calories: 661 kcal

Cheese Omelet

Preparation Time: 5 minutes

Cooking Time: 10 minutes

Servings: 2

Ingredients:

- 6 eggs
- 3 ozs. ghee
- 7 ozs. shredded cheddar cheese
- salt and pepper

Directions:

1. Whisk the eggs until smooth. Compound half of the cheese and season it with salt and pepper.
2. Melt the butter in a pan. Pour in the mixture and let it sit for a few minutes (3-4)
3. When the mixture is looking good, add the other half of the cheese. Serve immediately.

Nutrition: Carbs: 4 g Fat: 80 g Protein: 40 g Calories: 897 kcal

LUNCH

Buttered Cod

Preparation Time: 5 minutes

Cooking Time: 5 minutes

Servings: 4

Ingredients:

- 1 ½ lb. cod fillets, sliced
- 6 tablespoons butter, sliced
- ¼ teaspoon garlic powder
- ¾ teaspoon ground paprika
- Salt and pepper to taste
- Lemon slices
- Chopped parsley

Directions:

1. Mix the garlic powder, paprika, salt and pepper in a bowl.
2. Season cod pieces with seasoning mixture.
3. Add 2 tablespoons butter in a pan over medium heat.
4. Let half of the butter melt.
5. Add the cod and cook for 2 minutes per side.
6. Top with the remaining slices of butter.

7. Cook for 3 to 4 minutes.

8. Garnish with parsley and lemon slices before serving.

Nutrition: Calories 295 Total Fat 19g Saturated Fat 11g Cholesterol 128mg Sodium 236mg Total Carbohydrate 1.5g Dietary Fiber 0.7g Total Sugars 0.3g Protein 30.7g Potassium 102mg

Salmon with Red Curry Sauce

Preparation Time: 10 minutes

Cooking Time: 22 minutes

Servings: 4

Ingredients:

- 4 salmon fillets
- 2 tablespoons olive oil
- Salt and pepper to taste
- 1 ½ tablespoons red curry paste
- 1 tablespoon fresh ginger, chopped
- 14 oz. coconut cream
- 1 ½ tablespoons fish sauce

Directions:

1. Preheat your oven to 350 degrees F.
2. Cover baking sheet with foil.
3. Brush both sides of salmon fillets with olive oil and season with salt and pepper.
4. Place the salmon fillets on the baking sheet.
5. Bake salmon in the oven for 20 minutes.
6. In a pan over medium heat, mix the curry paste, ginger, coconut cream and fish sauce.
7. Sprinkle with salt and pepper.
8. Simmer for 2 minutes.
9. Pour the sauce over the salmon before serving.

Nutrition: Calories 553 Total Fat 43.4g Saturated Fat 24.1g Cholesterol 78mg Sodium 908mg Total Carbohydrate 7.9g Dietary Fiber 2.4g Total Sugars 3.6g Protein 37.3g Potassium 982mg

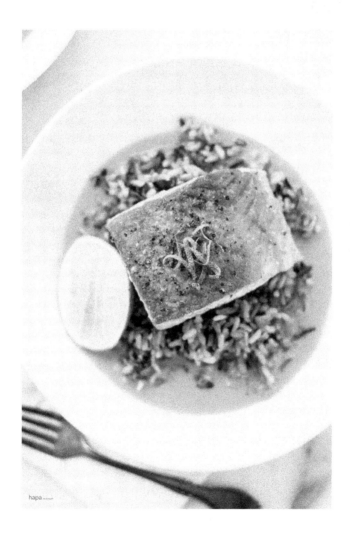

Salmon Teriyaki

Preparation Time: 15 minutes

Cooking Time: 25 minutes

Servings: 6

Ingredients:

- 3 tablespoons sesame oil
- 2 teaspoons fish sauce
- 3 tablespoons coconut amino
- 2 teaspoons ginger, grated
- 4 cloves garlic, crushed
- 2 tablespoons xylitol
- 1 tablespoon green lime juice
- 2 teaspoons green lime zest
- Cayenne pepper to taste
- 6 salmon fillets
- 1 teaspoon arrowroot starch
- ¼ cup water
- Sesame seeds

Directions:

1. Preheat your oven to 400 degrees F.
2. Combine the sesame oil, fish sauce, coconut amino, ginger, garlic, xylitol, green lime juice, zest and cayenne pepper in a mixing bowl.
3. Create 6 packets using foil.

4. Add half of the marinade in the packets.

5. Add the salmon inside.

6. Place in the baking sheet and cook for about 20 to 25 minutes.

7. Add the remaining sauce in a pan over medium heat.

8. Dissolve arrowroot in water, and add to the sauce.

9. Simmer until the sauce has thickened.

10. Place the salmon on a serving platter and pour the sauce on top.

11. Sprinkle sesame seeds on top before serving.

Nutrition: Calories 312 Total Fat 17.9g Saturated Fat 2.6g Cholesterol 78mg Sodium 242mg Total Carbohydrate 3.5g Dietary Fiber 0.1g Total Sugars 0.1g Protein 34.8g Potassium 706mg

Pesto Shrimp with Zucchini Noodles

Preparation Time: 10 minutes

Cooking Time: 15 minutes

Servings: 3

Ingredients:

- Pesto sauce
- 3 cups basil leaves
- ¾ cup pine nuts
- 2 cloves garlic
- ½ lemon, juiced
- 1 teaspoon lemon zest
- Salt to taste
- ¼ cup olive oil
- Shrimp and Zoodles
- 3 zucchinis
- Salt to taste
- 1 lb. shrimp
- 2 tablespoons avocado oil

Directions:

1. Put all the pesto ingredients in a blender.
2. Blend until smooth.
3. Spiralize the zucchini into noodle form.
4. Season with salt.

5. Drain water from the zucchini noodles.

6. Season the shrimp with salt and pepper.

7. Add half of the oil in a pan over medium heat.

8. Once the oil is hot, add the shrimp and cook for 1 to 2 minutes.

9. Add the remaining oil to the pan.

10. Add the zucchini noodles and cook for 3 minutes.

11. Add the pesto and toss to coat the noodles evenly with the sauce.

12. Season with salt.

Nutrition: Calories 304 Total Fat 22.2g Saturated Fat 2.6g Cholesterol 159mg Sodium 223mg Total Carbohydrate 8g Dietary Fiber 2.3g Total Sugars 2.5g Protein 21.3g Potassium 547mg

CONCLUSION

The things to watch out for when coming off keto are weight gain, bloating, more energy, and feeling hungry. The weight gain is nothing to freak out over; perhaps, you might not even gain any. It all depends on your diet, how your body processes carbs, and, of course, water weight. The length of your keto diet is a significant factor in how much weight you have lost, which is caused by the reduction of carbs. The bloating will occur because of the reintroduction of fibrous foods and your body getting used to digesting them again. The bloating van lasts for a few days to a few weeks. You will feel like you have more energy because carbs break down into glucose, which is the body's primary source of fuel. You may also notice better brain function and the ability to work out more.

Whether you have met your weight loss goals, your life changes, or you simply want to eat whatever you want again. You cannot just suddenly start consuming carbs again for it will shock your system. Have an idea of what you want to allow back into your consumption slowly. Be familiar with portion sizes and stick to that amount of carbs for the first few times you eat post-keto.

Start with non-processed carbs like whole grain, beans, and fruits. Start slow and see how your body responds before resolving to add carbs one meal at a time.

The ketogenic diet is the ultimate tool you can use to plan your future. Can you picture being more involved, more productive and efficient, and more relaxed and energetic? That future is possible for you, and it does not have to be a complicated process to achieve that vision. You can choose right now to be healthier and slimmer and more fulfilled tomorrow. It is possible with the ketogenic diet.

It does not just improve your physical health but your mental and emotional health as well. This diet improves your health holistically. Do not give up now as there will be quite a few days where you may think to yourself, "Why am I doing this?" and to answer that, simply focus on the goals you wish to achieve.

A good diet enriched with all the proper nutrients is our best shot of achieving an active metabolism and efficient lifestyle. A lot of people think that the Keto diet is simply for people who are interested in losing weight. You will find that it is quite the opposite. There are intense keto diets where only 5 percent of the diet comes from carbs, 20 percent is from protein, and 75 percent is from fat. But even a modified version of this which involves consciously choosing foods low in carbohydrate and high in healthy fats is good enough.

Thanks for reading this book. I hope it has provided you with enough insight to get you going. Don't put off getting started. The sooner you begin this diet, the sooner you'll start to notice an improvement in your health and well-being.